Chocolate Cake for the Thighs – The Anti-Diet Book for Women

101 FUN AND HELPFUL HEALTH & FITNESS TIPS

L. KAE GRANIEL

Bloomington, IN  Milton Keynes, UK

authorHOUSE®

AuthorHouse™
1663 Liberty Drive, Suite 200
Bloomington, IN 47403
www.authorhouse.com
Phone: 1-800-839-8640

AuthorHouse™ UK Ltd.
500 Avebury Boulevard
Central Milton Keynes, MK9 2BE
www.authorhouse.co.uk
Phone: 08001974150

First published by AuthorHouse 9/28/2006

ISBN: 1-4259-4203-2 (sc)

*Printed in the United States of America
Bloomington, Indiana*

This book is printed on acid-free paper.

A Special Thanks

I would like to take this space to thank my family and friends for supporting me whole heartedly in making this book a tangible reality. To my husband, who encouraged me to become a professional writer. To my daughters, Lex and Jaz, who entertained themselves so I could write in peace (most of the time). To my friendly editors Jennifer and Shari who labored over the content when I could no longer see the forest through the trees. And especially Donna, who's eagle eye for perfection gave it the final touch. Accomplishing anything without loved ones is difficult, to say the least. Mucho Mahalo and Aloha.

Foreword:

Diets don't work. If they did, no one would be overweight right? Take a moment to think about it. Let's just consider the way it sounds: DIEt. I think we can agree that it really does kill us to go on a DIEt or that we would rather die than go on one for any real length of time: am I right? OK, so how about the idea of just losing weight? Well, I personally don't like the idea of losing anything, it just sounds so stressful. Plus, it seems like as time goes by, all we do is actually find (and put on) the weight others have lost, plus some of our own. So, is there hope? Yes!

In 1981, I began the "yo-yo." By 1991, I had had enough. With a little observation, attention, journaling, and desire, I replaced a 177 lb. body with a 147 lb. one; moving out of a size 12 and into a size 8, and with the exceptions of two pregnancies, a broken ankle, and a mid-life crisis, have been there ever since. No pills, starvation, liquid meals, designer food, dry toast, or grapefruit!

This is not another weight loss / diet book. If anything, it is closer to a self help book. True, there is a lot of talk about food, but that's because there is a lot of talk about food in your day to day living. You will notice this book makes meal suggestions but never offers recipes. It makes reference to meal planning but never offers a meal plan. And nary' a tip mentions weighing & measuring food or counting calories. Instead, the focus is on making choices that move you in a positive way without extreme sacrifice.

Chocolate Cake for the Thighs was written from my pursuit of a happier, healthier, fitter mind and body. It's an enjoyable journey with great rewards. I urge you to modify or create your own tips to lead you on your personal quest. Over time, you will stay fit because your body wants to be that way. Eventually, your mind will think healthy thoughts. Together, your mind and body will create the image you desire and deserve. This may not happen overnight (although for some it may feel that way), or in 90 days, or a year. The truth is you'll never know when it happens. Because to be successful, you'll experience gradual, long lasting changes that become you. You will never "go off" this plan simply because you were never "on it" in the first place. From this moment on, you'll continue to reinvent your self and evolve to meet the needs of your ever changing life style. The changes you *choose to make* will not be difficult, just different. You will not give up anything you do not choose to.

The idea is simple. Start today with the small things you can do that make a difference (like walk after dinner) and see how quickly they positively affect and improve the way you look and feel. Before you know it, you'll actually be motivated to get rid of those bigger bad habits (like eating ice cream from the carton) by replacing them with new healthy ones.

The goal is not to be thinner. Losing weight will just be the icing on the cake when you pursue a healthier lifestyle that includes improvements in food choices, physical activity and mental support.

I do not claim to be a doctor, dietician, or psychologist. Not every tip is for everyone and some are just for laughs. What I do claim to be is a woman who finally chose to become healthy and fit. Today, I'm so passionate about my endeavor that I want to share it with the world. So here it is. I hope you enjoy it and it inspires you to become the truth of who you are. If you are so inspired, email me at lk@MindBodyLanguage. com and share your success or creative tips with me (I was already asked to make another collection). I would love to hear them.

Introduction

Just Say "NO" to the Yo-Yo.

Gaining and losing may be healthy and expected for the stock market, but not your body. The ups and downs of diets wreak havoc on your metabolism and mental health. "She's up, she's down, and she's big all around." Moderation is the biggest key to success in maintaining a healthy and fit body. Because this is not a diet, it will begin and continue with some introspection.

First things first; buy yourself a journal and ask yourself the following questions: #(1) Why do I want to lose weight? This may sound ridiculous but make an honest list, and if your main reason is to please some one other than yourself, forget it! #(2) At what weight will I look my best? _Not_ what do I want to weigh? There is a big difference between the thinnest we can remember being and a realistic everyday weight for our current lifestyle. #(3) What am I _willing_ to pay for my new healthier body. Remember, anything we actually _earn_ for ourselves means more than something briefly given. #(4) Why am I overweight? Get a legal sheet of paper and don't stop until you have filled every line with a specific reason, use two sheets if necessary. Avoid statements like "because I'm a pig or lazy". Those kinds of statements are cruel and damaging to your self-esteem, plus the fact that they are not specific. Try "because I drive through (fill in your favorite fast food place here) four to six times a week," or, "because I can eat a whole pint of ice cream in one sitting." Then tear off these sheets and fold them into your journal. Next, document _honestly_ how much your television is _on_ (**if you are watching or not**) for one whole week. This alone may be an alarming experience. Keep in mind that most people have conditioned themselves to eat in front of the T.V. So, all those TV hours equal lots of snacking.

Now, make a plan of action. Go back to that list and pick as many of the easy things you can and immediately remove them from your new and improved lifestyle (I started by eliminating all alcohol – except wine – and added one workout to my week). Try this easy stuff for a while, and when you've mastered those few, move on to more challenging ones (like eating fries only once a month). Time is on your side. The longer it takes to get rid of fat, the more likely you'll be able to keep it off, forever. Now here's the CHALLENGE. Are you ready? Maybe you should sit down. OK, no television for 21 days. I can hear your protests as to why you "have to watch." But listen; with very few exceptions (like home study T.V. courses) you can get anything you need from the radio (National Public Radio news), the internet, or newspaper in less time. And of course it wouldn't be a better lifestyle management program without exercise - but not necessarily *real exercise*. I suggest fake exercise like walking to the video store that is less than a ½ mile from your home to return movies (remember no T.V.) or unintentional exercise like mowing the lawn, bathing the cat, or shopping.

Then lastly, throw out your scale! You may weigh yourself once and only once. Write that number down on your calendar along with your measurements and make a solemn oath to never set foot on a scale for the rest of your life. Except of course at the doctor's where they don't even notice if you're wearing combat boots and holding a briefcase, or at the gym where you'll only stay on for a millisecond because you're petrified someone else might see the number. From this day forward your weight will be known to you only by the size of your clothes or the inches of a tape measure. I believe that weight is like age; it's all relative, and just a number. If this is too drastic for you, then go buy a digital scale that only works with a battery. Every time you weigh yourself take out the battery and put it away. This will remove the temptation to weigh often. The trouble with the scale is, as women, our weight can fluctuate dramatically when we are near and in our "cycle." This creates an inaccurate reading that can cause psychological damage. Another problem with the scale is the fact that if you have been "good" for the past few days and get on the scale and it shows a gain, you say "forget it" and give up and have some comfort food. But, if the scale shows a loss – even if it is just 1 pound – you decide you deserve a reward and go and eat something that is less than healthy. I know I've never clapped my hands after losing a couple of pounds and said, "Yippee, I'm going to indulge in some baby carrots with ranch."

This, my friends, is just the beginning. By accomplishing the aforementioned, you are now living; for the rest of your life, a better managed lifestyle full of rewards and benefits. Reading this book may burn a few calories, but it will not make you healthier or fit. Take action and allow yourself to feel excited about your adventure.

So, go on now and enjoy and embody the following 101 tips created to help you along your journey. Anytime you feel as though you're in a slump, sit down and evaluate your plan. Make adjustments and move on. Remember, to be successful, your plan must evolve to meet the needs of your current situation.

#1

Never eat ice cream out of the carton.

Or a cereal bowl. Use a teacup so one scoop seems like a lot.

Ice cream can actually have some really good ingredients and occasionally makes for a nice treat. Just remember that ice cream has four times as many calories when eaten out of the carton instead of a teacup. Why, because you eat four times as much. The psychology behind using the teacup is a visual one. A cereal bowl needs 3 to 5 scoops before it looks like a serving – especially if you like to pyramid it. Two scoops in a teacup however, are flowing over the rim and *looks* like a huge serving. You will find that you do not feel "gypped" out of those extra scoops – aka: calories. The other benefit to using a teacup is that when the ice crème melts, you can drink it!

#2

Make sure you "sea" salt.

If you must salt your food, switch to the more natural, less processed version – sea salt.

Remember, staying close to nature in your nutrition will lead to greater success with less effort. Many foods already come with a large dose of sodium. Sodium has been linked to hypertension and bloating. Too much salt will also make you thirsty and unfortunately, it may not be water you're drinking to quench that thirst. If you are not drinking water, you're drinking something with either a whole lot of calories or chemicals. Either way, it's not good.

Try pretending to shake salt on your food, seriously. Keep your salt shaker empty and just go through the motions – another psych that works. You'll notice that most of your food really tastes fine the way it is. And remember to get your iodine from another source. You could also buy reduced sodium salt as a first step.

#3

After eating frozen, prepared meals, eat the box they came in for roughage and trace minerals.

Seriously though, their true nutritional value is low and their sodium content is alarming.

The process of freezing and reheating food releases many of the naturally occurring vitamins, minerals, and antioxidants. Taste is also lost along with that nutrition, which is why sodium must be added in such large quantities. Frozen prepared meals are foods that can not remember where they came from. They're okay as an **occasional** "I'm in a hurry" meal. If you are choosing prepared meals that are made for the shelf (not frozen), keep in mind that various chemicals must be added to preserve shelf life and their packaging procedure also releases their nutrients.

#4

Keep veggie, fruit, and cheese pieces handy in your fridge.

This will help you make better food choices when you are starving or in a hurry.

Snacking and convenience go hand-in-hand. By having these items available in single serving sizes, you increase your chances of choosing something healthy for a snack, especially in the middle of the night. If you feel the urge for chips, try veggies with a dab of reduced fat ranch dip. Sometimes the crunchiness of fresh veggies can satisfy a chip craving, while the ranch can help with the salt and fat factors. If sugar is what you desire, fruits will always do the job because they're loaded with naturally occurring sugar (remember, even too much of natures sugar can be damaging). Cheese fills in nicely for fatty, greasy urges. When it comes to cheese, like sugar, too much can be just as bad as a bad food choice. Stick with white cheeses like Jack, Mozzarella, or Swiss. A slice of cheese in celery can conquer most cravings in a heartbeat. When possible, chop your cheese, fruit, and veggies yourself to help retain even more of that natural nutritional value. The precut, prepackaged items have often been a long time away from the farm/home.

#5

Always ask yourself, "is this the best food choice available to me right now?"

Sometimes your options are all unhealthy. And, sometimes you just gotta have some fries. No biggie, just make better choices next time and enjoy.

Pay attention to how often you somehow manage to get yourself into situations where there aren't any nutritional food choices and journal them. Better planning will help you in this area. Since convenience is the mother of fast food, start looking for what other quick but nutritional options may be at hand because they do exist, so seek them out.

When you go for the fries or cheesecake (don't be fooled by the word cheese), take a moment to think about something good you have done recently and remember that while you enjoy your indulgence. When you get down on yourself for eating junk food it creates a condition in which you will want junk every time you are feeling a bit down. Instead, turn your occasional junk food weakness into a chance to celebrate what a great person you are. Will you then create the urge to snack every time you feel good about yourself? YES, but as you begin to care more for yourself, you'll also desire to make better food choices – because you care. Make sense?

#6

Remember, you don't have to wait an hour before going into the water after you eat.

What a lame excuse for not working out if you have the chance. This is an old wives tale fabricated to give mothers the chance to eat their meal at a relaxed pace and clean up a little before they had to watch you in the water.

Anything is more comfortably accomplished when you allow your meal to digest a little. How long you need to digest depends upon what you ate and your personal digestive system.

Aqua exercise is one of the best non-impact fitness options available. Laps are OK, but try a group class too. The time goes by faster and motivation is easier to maintain when you're surrounded by others with a common goal.

#7

Never sit down with an entire bag or box of anything.

Especially if it's "family sized."

There is nothing worse that getting to the bottom of a big bag of chips and wondering how it happened – you were just going to have a few. Perhaps you may even make the excuse, "they don't fill them as much as they used to." Take a nice size portion or serving and put the bag or box away. It is rare that you'll feel cheated because you did not have the entire bag or box in one sitting.

#8

Always share your dessert. (and if you share with a man, you'll get less than half)

Unless of course you live alone, in which case you'll have to exercise portion control — sorry, or tell yourself you can only have dessert when a friend is visiting, or you dine out.

Dessert is one of life's simple pleasures and deserves *occasional* indulgence. If your meal does not feel complete without dessert, serve up some fruit instead, but slice it up and put it on a pretty saucer and eat it with a dessert fork — take advantage of the psychology of presentation. Ricotta cheese mixed with Splenda® and vanilla, or your favorite extract flavor can also satisfy that late sugar craving. (Stop making that face until you've tried it.) Desserts are the exception to occasionally consuming chemicals in the form of "fake sugar." And, of course, the Moderation Rule still applies.

#9

When a man (or one of your kids) asks while you're eating, "Are you going to eat all that or can I have it?" Let them have it.

No, I don't mean punch them.

Allow this to be the opportunity to check out your level of satiety. Perhaps you are actually already full (have reached satiety) but are enjoying the meal too much to give it up. In this case, either exercise self-control and give up your food anyway, or tell them "no" because you want the rest as your snack or, for lunch tomorrow.

The act of eating until we are stuffed is a problem many Americans suffer from and is a major contributor to obesity. Let this be the chance to exercise self control when it comes to eating. Keep in mind that if you prepared the meal, you probably have already eaten some while taste testing, so your serving should already be a little smaller when you sit down to eat.

Note: in my house, all leftovers are "open season" to the entire family after 24 hours.

#10

Watch out for mega milligrams of sodium.

Some processed, frozen meals, have over 300% of your recommended daily value of sodium – in one meal! Perhaps that's why the Pillsbury dough boy is so bloated – too much sodium.

When food is so far removed from its *organic* source and processed several ways to increase its shelf life, it loses not only nutrition, but taste. Sodium is added to give back some flavor, in addition to many other additives/chemicals. Find the time to care enough to eat foods with a higher nutritional/natural value.

#11

Choose between alcohol and dessert when dining out.

No cheating by choosing the Kahlua cheesecake or Rum cake!

The calorie count for a meal at most restaurants is through the ceiling. When you add alcohol **and** dessert, it goes off the Richter scale. Remember the key – moderation. What are you willing to pay for the body you claim to want?

#12

Forget the dishes. Go for a walk after dinner.

Sure, they'll still be there when you return, but now you'll have the energy to do them.

Actually, it would be even better to announce "I'm going for a walk, whoever chooses not to join me can do all the dishes." If you live alone, make this announcement anyway – just for fun. The less you feel like a walk, the more you need one.

Meals heavy in starchy or fatty foods cause the sleepy effect (insulin resistance) that can best be cured by natural "uppers" called endorphins. Endorphins kick into your system when you increase your heart rate and get oxygen rich blood. Plus, a lot of really nice conversation happens during a good walk. When you return, keep your "high" going by putting on the headphones and some kickin' music and attack those dishes with a little singing and dancing.

#13

It's time to lower your standards.

Look for "low" anything.
Low-cal, fat, salt, etc.

The goal is to not give up, but to improvise. Avoid *no* & *free* foods like no salt, fat free, or calorie free. The chemicals used to replace the calories and add flavor are unhealthy and your body has no use for them. Again with the moderation, you want to cut down – not out – your favorite foods.

Foods that are "reduced" often have a different flavor or texture. However, you will find some items that are just as good as, or even better than, the full on original. Try soy sauce with 50% less sodium and cream cheese with half the calories for starters. When it comes to food, think of yourself as a negotiator. Your role is to find what is best for all parties given the situation and circumstances.

#14

Replace the cream in your coffee with non-fat milk.

Because every little bit helps.

I know I just said "avoid no & free foods." But hey, there are exceptions to every rule. Besides, notice it's *not* called "no-fat" milk. That additional "n" totally changes the semantics. Seriously though, it's time to stop dragging your heels and walk with me on this one. Go through your daily food intake and look for opportunities to make little changes that can add up to big ones over time. Change is good. You are on a journey – remember?

#15

The cookie jar is not the place to take a stand.

Take a few and sit down.

Put some cookies on a plate or napkin. Then, before you sit down put back just one cookie. I guarantee you won't feel cheated. This also begins to train your mind and body to work together on your goal of a healthier, fitter body. You can do this with anything –like chips, fries or chocolate. After you have your serving, put back just a bit before you walk away. Oh, and remember to close the lid or put away the package after you serve yourself so you will not be tempted to have a few more when you put them away later.

#16

Turn off the T.V. while you eat.

Be in the moment, and relax and enjoy your meal.(If you have kids, never ask stressful questions like "so are you ready for the big test/game tomorrow?" Allow them to enjoy their meal too. Drama is for T.V. not dinner)

Tell funny or interesting stories. If you live alone and cannot stand the silence play a mellow CD. At least once a month, light some candles and eat with your best dishes. Like *Pavlov's Dogs* (who were conditioned to eat every time the bell rang), you condition yourself to eat every time you sit in front of the T.V. Even if you are not hungry, you will have the urge to snack. By keeping your T.V. off for 21 consecutive days, you can break that cycle and create a new habit where you actually pay attention to what and how much you are eating.

Having the T.V. off also allows you to relax, (which aids in proper digestion) and be grateful for your meal. A few moments of gratitude every day will noticeably improve the quality of your life because you will receive more of that which you focus on. So take the time at every meal (or snack) to focus on all that you do have to be thankful for – no matter how small – instead of what you don't have. Begin now to get more of what you want.

#17

Never eat in the living room.

You are less likely to lie around for hours after you eat when you eat at the dining room table.

In this case it would even be better to stand at the counter or over the sink and eat. If you live alone or don't have a dining room table, then buy a sturdy stand up tray and eat facing out a window, on your patio, or in another room with some nice music playing. If you're eating in the living room, you are probably slouching – which hampers proper digestion, or even worse, watching T.V. Watching the news while eating also creates a negative conditioning with eating which leads to eating every time things aren't going to well for you.

#18

Keep your life simple
& your meals complex.

Especially when it comes to carbs.

Carbohydrates fuel the body and feed the brain. So why do they have such a bad rap? Because the truth is, if you want to lose weight fast, eliminating carbs is the fastest way to do it. We all know that when we reduce our caloric intake enough and exercise more, our body will burn fat to fuel our body – resulting in weight loss. Since carbs break down into "fuel" faster and easier than fat, some believe that carbs are bad because they get in the way of fat burning. Plus, unused carbs are nothing but fat waiting to happen.

Here is the truth. Eliminating carbs is dangerous. Your body is not designed to constantly burn fat for fuel. Without carbs you will experience varying levels of light headedness, absent mindedness, and fatigue. Many people also experience depression and mood swings. Too many simple carbs cause something known as insulin resistance, where the body can not properly process fuel so it ends up as fat around the midsection – for starters. So what's a girl to do? Think complexity and M-O-D-E-R-A-T-I-O-N.

Carbs 101 – there are basically two kinds of carbohydrates, simple & complex. Simple carbs are the ones that breakdown quickly and easily. Think starch and you've nailed most of the simple carbs. Most potatoes, pasta, baked goods, and chips fall into this category. Since it's difficult to only consume the recommended ½ cup serving size of these foods – they are trouble. Indulging in more than a ½ cup serving at any meal forces the insulin resistance issue and impairs the body's natural ability to metabolize effectively (burn calories).

Complex carbs are your friend. They are closer to nature with all their fiber and pulp. During digestion, fiber helps slow down the release of glucose (sugar) found in carbs which allows the body to kick in an accepted amount of insulin. This eliminates the insulin resistance issue. Complex carbs are fruits, vegetables, and whole grains. But even these friendly carbs have issues. If they are super sweet like cantaloupe, pineapple, corn, and carrots – use moderation. Apples, berries, legumes, and sweet potatoes are better choices. And remember to seek out whole (not refined) wheat, multigrain, and high fiber starches. As a rule of thumb, the grams of fiber on the label should be 4g or higher.

#19

Accept no substitutes.

Your body knows how to process calories, not chemicals.

Like most things in life, it's a little bit give and take. When it comes to food however, substitutions are not your friend. The amount of chemicals that go into our processed food is alarming. Why are we so surprised that cancers are claiming more and more lives every year, even the lives of healthy people who never smoked. It's the chemicals folks. And this is no conspiracy theory. An old friend of mine used to work for a big cola company. His job was to service the fountains around town. When I was considering switching to diet sodas – to help me lose weight of course – he had me meet him at one of his stops. My friend, out of care for my future health, showed me what happens to the rubber rings of the diet soda canisters. I was shocked. Not only were the rings eaten alive, but he told me how they get that way every 2 or 3 months. Remember the shocking news about cancer and saccharin? Come on folks, this is just common sense. Our bodies store those unfamiliar chemicals in our bodies until they pile up into a polluted wasteland that eventually wreaks havoc.

Look for foods that are processed *low* or *reduced* instead of replaced. Low-fat milk, reduced fat peanut butter, and lower sodium spam are a few examples. And as always, choose to eat foods that can remember where they came from – remembering to wash those fruits & veggies.

#20

Try a "veggie burger" or make Tofu parmesan.

It won't kill you to step out of the box. They are actually way better than they sound.

If you want to make lasting changes you'll need to replace old habits with new ones. Expanding your dietary preferences will help sustain long term change. It's time to play around with and rearrange your food options.

If you must eat frozen meals, try a veggie burger. They vary greatly in taste so ask a vegetarian friend to suggest a brand or read the ingredients and choose one that sounds okay. Melt a slice of jack, muenster, or swiss cheese on top to help make it more familiar. Eat it on a wheat bun with your favorite burger toppings. If you're a die hard carnivore, add a tablespoon of chili con carne on top.

Tofu is awesome because it absorbs the flavor of whatever you cook it with. Marinara and soy sauce are especially good. Tofu is your friend because it is high in protein without the fat. So experiment with it and create tofu tacos, lasagna, chow mien or chocolate pudding (OK perhaps not the pudding – but hey, I'm gonna' try it now).

Note: only experiment with new healthy dishes when you have some leftovers in the fridge - just in case it's really bad. I once made scalloped sweet potatoes – they tasted sooo much better in my imagination.

#21

When you have the urge to snack, grab some nuts.

Get your mind out of the gutter.

Nuts got a bad rap because they are often high in fat. But we're talking "natures" (unsaturated) fat here people. Moderation says, just eat a big handful. Remember, your body knows what to do with naturally occurring fat vs. saturated fat. Nuts are a great snack choice because they are crunchy with protein and natural fat, all of which have a lasting effect on ridding hunger pangs and sugar highs/lows. Some nuts are healthier than others, but the truth is, any nuts are better than a bag of chips. Watch out for salted, toffee, honey, or chocolate covered nuts – silly goose.

#22

Give a list of your bad food habits to your kids and tell them you're not allowed to eat them any more.

Hear how great your loving advice sounds when it comes back at you from the mouth of your kids.

You'll learn a lot about how you parent when you give your children the power. This tip is only for people who *really* want to rid themselves of bad food choices. It works very well if you have the will power to smile and hug your child every time they catch or correct you. If you ever snap at them for helping you, this tip is over.

#23

Get lipo-sucked.

But remember, unless you are working out and making better food choices, the new fat has to go somewhere, and it isn't ever where you want it to go.

In some cases bariatric surgery is necessary. But for many Americans, the procedure is strictly cosmetic. The problem is - surgery does nothing to change your habits/diet. If you thought fat on your belly and thighs looked bad, wait till you see it show up with the same intensity on your back, around your knees, and hanging from your jaw line.

For those of you who had cosmetic surgery and were so motivated by the change, you changed your lifestyle to support your new look indefinitely – I applaud you. You are the exception rather than the rule. So, if you're considering liposuction, make sure you have a healthy and fit lifestyle <u>first</u> so that you benefit permanently from your sacrifice.

#24

Get an herbal body wrap.

It's only temporary but great for special occasions like weddings and high school reunions.

Spa body wraps can actually take several inches off your belly, butt, and thighs. Some even help detoxify the body and leave you feeling better. They are generally somewhat expensive so ask for one as a gift. A good pampering at a spa always helps a gal feel and look better, even if it is just for a day.

#25

If you must weigh yourself daily, make one ounce a day your weight loss goal.

Steady and slow is the best way to go.

To weigh in ounces you will need a digital scale. After you get tired of the ups and downs of daily weighing, take out the battery and only weigh yourself once a month on whatever number happens to be your birthday number – like the 11th. It's natural for the body to "flat line" during weight loss as it adjusts to the new lifestyle so be patient and keep on keeping on because it won't last forever. Since the body functions in cycles, it is possible to not lose weight for 3 weeks or even 3 months at a time. This is the ideal time to **switch to the tape measure** or mix up your dietary choices and workout regime (or start a workout regime!)

Hello!

Just thought I'd mention that you are a quarter of the way through this book. Did you buy a journal? Have you taken any notes to help you remember what you read? Did you already make your list for change? Did you make that list of bad food habits for your kids? If you're reading this purely for entertainment, please excuse the interruption. However, if you're reading it to become fit and healthy, then go back and read the intro again and put some changes into action. Too much information can be overwhelming. It's better to take it in stages. Okay, go now – the rest will be here when you return (I promise)..

#26

Get a haircut; shave your legs & armpits, and get a bikini & brow wax.

That ought to be good for a few ounces off on the scale, or more depending upon your nationality.

This is a silly example of the extremes some people will go to lighten the load on the scale. Like many quick fixes, it's only temporary – unless you have decided to make these activities part of your daily life. I wonder how many calories shaving your legs actually burns? It should at least qualify as a workout with all that bending and twisting

#27

Whenever possible, eat your lunch "topless."

You know…when you order a sandwich without the top bread. Some call it open faced but it's called "topless" in my neck of the woods. Besides, it got your attention didn't it?

This is a perfect example of something simple you can do to save yourself from a few empty calories. You can also eat a burger this way when you put the lettuce on top instead of the bun. And you can go even one better by eliminating the bread all together. Try these for starters: (1) wrap your burger and all it's fixin's in a big leaf of dark green lettuce; (2) put your taco meat into a crispy cabbage leaf; (3) roll your cheese and meat in a big floppy lettuce leaf instead of a tortilla. These are easy ways to move your meal from simple to complex. (see tip #18)

#28

Take all the clothes that don't fit you any more out of your closet – and donate them!

They'll be out of style by the time they fit again anyway. Or at least you'll deserve a shopping spree for your new hard earned body.

Warning: this is a chick tip.

Keeping clothes that do not fit you in your closet is ill advised for several reasons: #(1) It makes you think you have more clothes than you do which causes problems when you really need a special something to wear and you have nothing. This leads to throwing yourself on your bed in a fit of depression which usually leads to a pig out. #(2) When you have "fat & skinny" clothes in your closet, you can keep in living the yo-yo (no no). The ups and downs of the yo-yo body are dangerous for your emotional and physical health. When you're in your "skinny" clothes you feel great. But there is that voice reminding you not to get used to it because, "you know you can't stay this way." Then, when you are in your "fat" clothes you're depressed because you know you could be thinner. Getting thin usually means going on some diet that keeps you from eating regular healthy foods ("lose weight the natural way by eating nothing but fruit" PLEASE or "start your day with eggs and a ½ pound of bacon & you wont be hungry till dinner" HELLO heart disease). It's time for a déjà vu. Diets don't work – if they did, people would not be overweight. #(3) A closet full of clothes in a variety of sizes keeps you from really evaluating what size is appropriate for a healthy mind and body – at this time.

Now is the time to think "fit" vs. "thin." Remove all those unwearable clothes (no matter how desirable) and choose a size that is appropriate for today. Take a look at yourself in a full length mirror and be grateful for the body you currently have because the truth is, it could be bigger. Imagine someone you know who is bigger than you – somehow it is usually a relative – and again feel gratitude for the body you are currently in. Yeah it could be better but right now we're focusing on being grateful for all that we do have. Look at your body and know that you are HOT. Seriously, there are many men out there who would take you in a minute if you just gave them the chance. Of course the problem is, we never want the ones that want us – why is that ladies? Anyway, sexy is state of mind, not a size (think Mae, Star, and Anna Nicole). Now clean out that closet!

Inventory what you have and need in your journal. Then, take yourself to a discount store or big sale and buy yourself a few things to update your look. Don't be foolish and spend hundreds of dollars on clothes that you may only be *passing* through. But none the less, buy nice things that fit well and look nice. Remember to love your current body while trying on clothes and be <u>complimentary</u> and <u>supportive</u> with your comments to yourself.

#29

Aim for the size in which you look your best. NOT the smallest size you can remember wearing.

Notice we are talking size here, not weight.

It's hard for me not to slap the woman who says, "I don't understand, I used to wear a 6 when I graduated high school." I don't want to slap them because I am jealous or because I am mean. I want to slap them to change their state and bring them into this decade. Back then, they probably also lived at home, earned $2.95 an hour, and paid 39 cents a gallon for gas. All of that was then, and this is now. Times have changed and so have you. Perhaps you have had children or have been exposed to something called stress. The fact is, you are now a woman and it is time to aim for the size a woman would wear, not a 17 year old girl. If you happen to get back into that size six, great as long as you look healthy and fit. Not saggy, starved, and skinny.

As women, we are genetically smart. This means we instinctually know at what size we look our best. There is a certain general weight and specific size we know we're meant to be. When we are there, we look and feel great. This is the size we're striving for now. It may take a while to get there – remember, no more yo-yo. So enjoy the journey because you know where you are going and that knowledge should feel really good.

#30

Don't watch your weight.
Watch your plate.

Treat the cause, not the symptom.

Watching your weight is not helpful because the scale can do nothing to make you lighter. Watch your plate – or more importantly, your hands, because they do the real snacking. When we begin to choose healthy foods that are unrefined and closer to their natural state, our body responds by looking and feeling better. I'm not talking about tofu milkshakes and bean sprouts sandwiches on 9 grain bread, so stop it. I am talking about eating more of what we enjoy that we know is good for us, and less of what we enjoy that we know is bad for us. Shift the balance of power to healthier foods and watch them win the battle of the bulge for you.

Don't force yourself to eat stuff you don't enjoy because life is too short to eat yucky stuff. I for one, refuse to eat bell peppers or bread that weighs more than my purse. You on the other hand, may love bell peppers and heavy bread – so go for it. The point is, it's time to stop being so childish and time to expand what we are willing to try. Because our pallet changes as we grow older, the odds are good that we can now enjoy foods we used to hate as kids (for me it's beets). So give the good stuff a chance and see what happens.

#31

Whenever you get the urge to snack, turn on Rap (or Classical) music.

This will create a negative conditioning to snacking.

As much as music can be a motivator, it can be an irritant. My sincerest apologies if I suggested a genre of music you happen to love. The idea is for you to fill in the blank and play whatever music it is that gets under your skin, and play it loudly. If you're one of those people who claim to love every type of music, try *talk* radio.

Pick something you can't stand and remember to play it loudly. Keep it on until you are no longer thinking about snacking and have come up with something else to do – unless of course you choose watching T.V. You were probably already watching T.V. in the first place and that's why you felt the urge to snack. Remember, T.V. has that effect on most people. (Re-read #16 & #17)

#32

Join a gym, health or country club, and actually go.

Join with a friend and increase you chances of working out regularly.

Learn to put your self/health first, because it is the right thing to do. I am currently a fitness instructor (only 3 classes a week). Now wait, don't go saying "oh you're one of those people." The truth is, I teach fitness classes because I found out the hard way that if I was not "required" to be there – I simply didn't go. It is so hard to find the time to workout. You're either tired, hungry, have errands, or don't like the class offered at the time you can workout. What I found out was, in teaching, I still got everything done because I had to. And, because I was working out I felt better, had more energy, and was happier about doing it.

Fact: working out kicks in endorphins which cause a natural state of increased stamina and happiness.

I'm sure the real reason why you have not joined a club yet is because you have a **really big but.** You know, like "I would join **but** I don't have the time, or **but** I'd feel uncomfortable, or **but** I can't really afford it." The time has come to put your big but aside and join.

It would be great if you worked out anywhere. Clubs offer things you just can't get at home or in a park, like childcare and group energy. Did you know that you can put your "rug rats/darlings" in childcare at most clubs for about $2 a kid for 2 hours of workout time? Imagine the bliss of 2 child free hours. Many women at my club workout for 1 hour then shower & change, and meet for coffee at the club snack bar for another ½ hour. Do this 3 times a week and working out will soon be your priority. If you can't afford it, then start looking at all the money you're spending on your kids and cut back just enough to afford what you need. I know you know it's possible.

Now, choosing a club is the hard part. Here are the guidelines: (1). Make sure it is close to things that you do so you can drop by easily. (2). Make sure they offer child care (if applicable). (3). (go for free on a pass for a week or month) Look at the schedule and make sure you can choose at least 3 classes a week you like at times you can go. (4). Never join at full price. All clubs offer "no initiation/enrollment fee" specials all the time. If you can afford it, sign up for one personal training session, but instead of working out a plan spend your hour having them teach you how to use all the cardio equipment and weight machines. A big fear in going to the gym is looking silly. When you join with a friend you can stand there together and figure things out or giggle together when you bump into each other during a class. Of course you can always ask some one else how to use those machines. Most women would be happy, happy, happy to help you out. So allow for their happiness and ask. (If you live in a rural area you may have to join community recreation classes – so go ahead and do it – today!)

#33

Shot put your scale.

It'll be good exercise — but warm up first.

Weighing yourself daily is a sadistic habit. If your weight is up, you get depressed and eat. If your weight is down, you reward your self with a little something/snack. Either way it leads to comfort food. "Just say no to the yo-yo."

(Read the introduction and # 25 again) If you must weigh, go buy a digital scale that only works with a battery. Every time you weigh yourself take out the battery and put it away. This will remove the temptation to weigh often. Only weigh once a month and write that number on the calendar. Oh, and always weigh naked, first thing in the morning, after you have gone potty, and removed all jewelry, contact lenses, or glasses.

#34

Measure your weight only by a tape measure or how your clothes fit.

Go back and read the intro, #25 and #33.

There are five measurements you need to be concerned with

1. thigh

2. butt

3. belly

4. waist

5. back

Measure your thigh at the widest part and straight around. Be careful that the tape measure does not angle up or down the thigh. With your feet together, measure your butt around the biggest part. The belly button is usually the widest part of your belly, if not, measure around the widest part. Your waist is measured around the smallest part between your hips and the bottom of your ribcage – not necessarily where you wear your pants. And your back is measured right below your boobs (pick them up and out of the way if necessary). We are more concerned with your back fat than bust line.

When you work out *you will weigh more* as your muscles eliminate the fat and become tone and dense. The scale will show weight gain – which is depressing – while the real story is - **you're slimming down and getting fit!** A tape measure will tell the true story as fat is burned away by the muscle. Women do not bulk when they work out so don't even go there. And besides, would you rather be bulky with fat or muscle?

The healthiest and easiest way to check your weight is to put on your jeans 3 times a week. Actually have a pair that fit well (without Lycra) to use for this purpose. Never actually wear those jeans around. They have become your new scale – and you wouldn't wear your scale out, would you? If you wear them, you'll have to wash them, and more importantly, DRY them. We all know what freshly dried jeans can do to our image ego. Now if your "scale jeans" ever fit like they have just come out of the dryer, it is time to look at your lifestyle and make some simple but immediate changes. And, when your "scale jeans" become baggy – meaning the waist is at least 2 inches too big – go out a buy a new pair, and give the old pair to charity because there is no going back. If however, you have lost 2 inches off your waist because you were on a diet of some sort, keep those jeans, because you will be that size again as soon as you go off the diet so there is no sense in wasting $40. Oh, come on – it's the truth and you know it. If there was a diet that worked, you would not be reading this book. Diets only work if you commit yourself to eating that way for the rest of your life. There hasn't been a diet designed that makes exceptions for celebrations, vacations, set backs, relocations, in town guests, out of town work, pregnancy, bouts of depression, and menopause (in other words, life). So, shot put that scale and make lifestyle changes that include working out and making better food choices. These are things you can continue to do no matter what life throws your way.

#35

Eat before you eat.

Say what?!

There are several situations in which you should eat before you eat: # (1) whenever it has been more than 3 hours since your last meal/snack. "I don't want to ruin my appetite for dinner by having a snack now" – WRONG. When you are feeling famished, you'll be more likely to overeat or load up on the simple carbs because your body knows that's the quickest way to calories; # (2) before you go out to a party where they will be serving lots of fattening and not so healthy stuff. Buffets are a good example of this; #(3) if you know in advance you will not be liking the food served there. Sometimes people are bad cooks, use ingredients we don't like, or too much grease. Some restaurants are not your favorite, or perhaps you are vegetarian and your food choices are too limited; and # (4) you do not know when you will be eating again. Many events don't serve the food at the time stated – if a time was even stated at all. This leads to having alcohol on an empty stomach (because the alcohol is ALWAYS being served), which always spells T-R-O-U-B-L-E.

Eating a bit before you eat in these situations will reduce grouchiness, and help keep you stabilized. Of course the snacks you choose to eat before you eat will be healthy (review tip #4) or else you are just doubling up the empty calories.

#36

Remember, to be forever, it should take at least twice as long to lose weight as it did to gain it.

It doesn't happen over night either way.

Steady and slow is the way to go. Just say no to the yo-yo (getting tired of hearing that yet?) When you make gradual changes, it is easier for your mind and body to get on board. Change is scary, and in the caveman days, usually led to death. Today, exactly the opposite is true. Stress is caused by the lack of ability to change. You will live longer and healthier when you learn how to manage and embrace change (easier said than done – I know). So stick with it. Don't give up so easily. Find someone you can confide in. Someone who will remind you to stick with it because it's the right thing to do and there is light at the end of the tunnel.

Supposedly, it takes 21 days to make a permanent behavioral change, so commit yourself to sticking with whatever you started. You must have thought it was possible or you never would have started it to begin with. I for one would never give up cheese or take up jogging because I know I couldn't stick with it. Make realistic choices and believe in yourself because as the saying goes, "anything believed is easily achieved."

#37

Avoid the grocery store when hungry or depressed.

You know that.

<u>Problem:</u> Knowing and doing are often two different things. We lead hectic lives and often have to shop when we are hungry because there is nothing at home to eat. Hello!! The trouble comes with what we put into our cart when we feel famished or are seeking comfort food. I once bought a box of something like a Ho-Ho® that was also laced with caramel and within 5 days had eaten the entire box (of course two were gone before I even got home).

<u>Solution:</u> As soon as you enter the store, go to the section that sells party platter stuff (staying away from the brownie squares – of course). Pick out a small container of your favorite fruit, deviled eggs, or cheese cubes and eat that while you shop. Yep, open it up right there in your cart and feast away. Stay to the perimeter of the isles and shop until at least 10 minutes has passed and your blood sugar has stabilized. All the healthy stuff is usually around the edges of a store. By then you should feel normalized and it is now safe to enter the bowels of the store where they keep the snacks and frozen foods. Make sure you keep the container of what you ate and pay for it when you check out.

You can also delegate the shopping to someone else. Make a list and send them on their way. It is true they will not buy the right size, brand, or quantity, and they won't have enough sense to buy things they know you need but are not on the list.

This is OK. At least most of the shopping will be done and that will free you up to go work out. In order to be successful at most things, you will have to give up some control and the notion that only you can do it right and delegate (please read the previous sentence again – slowly – then digest it and become it).

As far as depression goes, try shopping on Saturday morning, right after breakfast, before you have time to get depressed about anything. Since working out is the death of depression, avoid the store and go to the gym instead. Then after you workout, go shopping. If you're starving by then, go to the party platter section and make your choice.

#38

Walk the dog – or your husband – everyday, and twice on weekends.

You both deserve it.

If you don't have dogs or a man (count your blessings – just kidding☺ dogs are good for you), that's OK, just walk yourself right after dinner (remember tip #12?). Walking the dogs at least once a day can also help eliminate many canine behavior problems. Walking your self is good for digestion and will boost your stamina. When possible, walk with someone. Social interaction is good for us, and like the dogs, it helps eliminate behavioral problems. If you're walking alone, put on headphones and listen to music that moves you. No talk radio because the goal is to get motivated not irritated. Most talk radio is confrontational or frustrating, and those are two states you definitely want to avoid after a meal – or any time for that matter.

You have three opportunities a day to walk. If you're not the early bird (5 am) type, then walk at lunch with a co-worker or after dinner as mentioned. Walking is another way to kill the munchies. Simply walk out the door the next time to feel the urge to snack. I promise, by the time you return, the urge will be gone. If it isn't, you did not walk long enough. When you start to feel really happy, energized, and/or like a winner, your endorphins have kicked in and your mission accomplished.

#39

Take a dance class.

Meet muscles you never knew you had.

Most cities and towns have a community center or a parks and recreation. Go on down and sign up for that class you've always wanted to take. Ballet, ballroom, salsa, or line-dancing are all good choices. These classes are usually inexpensive and do not require a long term commitment. If you are serious about getting fit, sign up for a dance class at your community college. Who knows, you may find yourself in their upcoming production of West Side Story (OK, maybe not). You do not need a partner. Although, it would be helpful to sign up with a friend so you have someone to laugh and carpool with.

If you hate gyms, this is the choice for you. If you're afraid, sign up anyway. I'll bet you'll find yourself in a room full of people who are as scared as you. Be fore warned however, there are "professional amateurs" in every class. They are the ones who show up in costume. This is their hobby – judge them not – for one day "they" could be "you." OK, maybe not.

#40

Talk about it.

*At least **talking** about losing weight burns more calories than just **thinking** about it.*

What? It's true. Talking is also good because then you'll have to walk your talk and we all know how good walking is for you. Your word is your wand, where it goes, so do you.

So go ahead, start telling people how you've decided to get fit and make better food choices – I double dare ya!

#41

Buy new aerobic shoes.

*They put such a spring in your step
you'll feel like you've lost 10 pounds.*

Make sure you invest in good shoes – not cute ones. Sometimes you get lucky and find good cute ones, but this will not be the goal when shopping for a new pair. Buying fitness shoes today can be daunting. The choices are overwhelming. So here are your guidelines.

#1 Buy shoes that suit your chosen activity. Walking and running shoes should have strong heel support and shock absorbency. These shoes are designed to support the foot as it rolls forward from heel to toe. Running shoes are terrible for fitness classes because they don't allow for quick movement in multiple directions which will take its toll on your ankle. If you decided to join a gym, you'll need what they call studio shoes. Studio shoes are more flexible (less stiff) than running shoes. They should have heel and forefoot support, as well as extra stitching for lateral (side to side) movement. Studio shoes are usually good for any fitness class or cardio machine (like the treadmill). Studio shoes are also called aerobic or cross-trainer shoes. These shoes are terrible for running because they do not absorb enough shock. If you can, try and find mid-top aerobic shoes to add extra protection in lateral movements. AVIA has the best mid-top aerobic shoes on the market. In my personal experience, AVIA makes the best fitness shoes because they put function before fashion. It seems as though they spend more money on research, design, and development, than marketing. If you can find them, buy the 681. Try their website (and no I am not getting paid for this endorsement, it's just that when you find something good you want to share it). Nike makes a shoe called Nike-free that feels like a ballet slipper with support. You can actually fold it in half. I like this shoe a lot too. It's also a mid-top but the Velcro strap won't stay strapped once you start moving. And I should also mention that RYKA is a company founded by a woman who knows women's feet. RYKA also donates money from the sale of every shoe to women's cancer research. Check out their website also. Note: Sorry I have zero experience with running shoes. I never choose jogging for working out. I do not like it – it hurts. I only run when being chased. I know people who LOVE to run, they tell me if I run long enough I'll get the "runner's high" that makes it all worth it. I prefer the group energy of a fitness class. So to each her own because whatever your choice, it's all good! *We like to move it, move it.*

#2 Buy shoes that fit right. Make sure you have on the right socks on when buying your fitness shoes. I don't have to tell you what a good fit feels like. Ladies always know a good fit when they feel it. It's just that sometimes we'll choose a shoe because of price or cuteness. Rule of thumb – if the shoe is super cute, it's probably a crappy fitness shoe. Good fitness shoes look just like that – a good fitness shoe. And besides, once you buy your fitness shoes, NEVER wear them around town. They are to be used strictly for the fitness activity you chose them for. This is very important. If you wear your shoes around town they will stretch out in the wrong way and wear out sooner. If they are a studio shoe, they will get ugly. Buy those cute tennies for running around town. If you're using them 5 times a week, expect to buy new fitness shoes every 4 to 6 months because they stretch out and break down. Or, find good insoles (I like Happy Feet insoles with arch support) and just replace them one time and buy new shoes next time to help save money.

#3 Buy shoes that are on sale. Of course. All shoes go on sale – you know that. I am strongly against charging things you can't afford to pay cash for. However, this is the exception. You need good shoes to work out in and you need them now. If you can't afford it – charge it. Put yourself first and get those shoes. Remember, we're only talking one pair ladies, not three or four. If you are going to jog **and** go to the gym you will need two pairs. But that sounds like a bit much for starters.

#42

Wear all black.

It's very slimming.

It's true – enough said.

#43

When people ask if you are on a diet, tell them "no" you are just eating right.

Because the truth shall set you free.

We may be turning our backs on dieting forever, but are still keeping a close eye on our diet. Diet actually means whatever it is that you eat regularly. Choosing not to eat is the worst choice of all. So take a moment and look at your diet. Think about what healthy and fit improvements you could make and make them happen.

Remember, *diet* now means how you normally eat on a regular basis, not eating less or weird. And, if you are drinking a meal, you are not on the path to health and fitness. How weird is the term "meal replacement?" It sounds so "Logan's Run" (sorry for dating my self) It may help if you understand Ectomorphs, Mesomorphs, and Endomorphs, and what diet is best for them.

The Ectomorph (morph means body) is the body that has boundless, often fidgety energy. The Ectomorph has trouble keeping weight on and actually loses weight around the holidays. Stress causes them to lose weight. Ectomorphs have a naturally fast metabolism (the rate at which they burn calories). This means that they often crave caffeine, sugar and starch (which digests into a quick sugar fix) to keep them fueled. This is the person you know who eats doughnuts and candy and is thin as a rail. But being thin and being fit are two different things. To become fit, if you are the Ectomorph, you must workout daily and choose complex carbohydrates like fruit & brown rice over candy and pasta. Sugar makes an already fast metabolism even crazier. So choose foods that are slower in digestion and watch you body respond in a healthy way.

The Mesomorph is the body that gains weight the moment you stop working out. When you were young you could eat whatever you wanted and never had to worry about your weight. Mesomorphs always weigh more than they look like they weigh because they carry more muscle weight. If you are a Mesomorph, as you mature, your metabolism slows down and you gain weight more easily. In order to be healthy and fit, you must workout daily and eat smart. Over time you should notice that you get full easier. Stop eating when you feel even a little bit full and save the rest for another meal. Because your body has grown accustomed to performing your favorite sport (all Mesomorphs play a sport) you'll have to cross train to get the body you desire. As long as you stay active and don't over indulge in junk food, your body will look and feel great.

The Endomorph is the body that seems to gain weight just looking at food. Endomorphs have always been "chubby." The good news is Endomorphs tend to be less prone to stress, can be more easy going and enjoy life more. On the inside, unless they are obese, the Endomorph is the healthiest with the steadiest metabolism. Unfortunately, it is steady at a slower rate. Working out has to be a priority for the Endomorph because over time they are most likely to become dangerously obese. Actually, just an active life style and a career that keeps you moving can be helpful. If you happen to be an Endomorph, you must choose foods that digest slowly like vegetables, fruit, and grains. And remember to stop eating the moment you feel full. Find a workout you really enjoy and stick with. Stay faithful to your veggies and you can keep obesity at bay, living healthy, happy and fit.

#44

Remember, it's not the calories, it's the contents that count.

An avocado half is better for you than a handful of chips with the same calorie count.

Think *quality* not *quantity*. Choose foods that your body knows how to use. Naturally occurring sugar and fat digest and metabolize steadier than refined and processed ones. Making the healthy choice allows you to avoid those energy highs and lows and assists in eliminating that overwhelming desire for a three o'clock nap. Consider yourself precious and eat foods that are valuable. A list of precious, semi-precious, and rhinestone foods can be found at the end of the book. (Go ahead and peek now – You know you want to)

Moderation, as always is the key to success here. More of a good thing is not the idea. Eating an entire avocado, half pound of nuts, or container of hummus will eventually push you out of the size you are currently wearing. Just because they are good for you does not mean they are calorie free. Use common sense and eat a reasonable serving.

#45

Don't think you're making a healthy food choice because the package of "Red Vines" says "Fat Free" in the corner.

You know better than that!
It may truly be fat-free, but that does not mean it won't make you fat.

Refined sugar and starches are probably the reason why you are overweight. The sooner you cut them back, the sooner you'll be seeing that body you so desire. Replacing them with fruit and other complex carbs is a good first step.

Note: I am not saying you can never have sugary treats, pasta, potatoes, or chips. I am saying, "it's time to cut back" – way back. Begin with smaller servings and switching to complex carbs like wheat pasta (stop making that face). Fiber is your friend – also in moderation of course. Look for 4g or higher on the food label (review tip #18 again).

#46

Remember, No-fat or No-salt, usually means No-flavor (but added chemicals).

*Seek out **reduced** and **less** when shopping.*

Foods that are *reduced* and *less* add up to a reduced and less you. I once tried sodium free green beans. They were so horrible that even putting sea salt on them didn't help. And although fat free milk is a good thing, I can't handle it. It reminds me of when we were poor and drank powdered milk. I do enjoy bacon with 50% less salt, reduced fat mayo, and jelly with 25% less sugar – to name a few. So go ahead and play around with all the *reduced* and *less* options there are available to you. Find what you like, make the switch and begin getting fit.

#47

Every time you get the urge to snack, brush your teeth.

Seriously

Go out and buy yourself a **soft** bristle tooth brush. Brushing your teeth whenever you have the urge to snack keeps you from snacking for two reasons. #1 Psychologically, brushing implies that you have already eaten. This fools the brain by using conditioning; much like how always snacking in front of the TV causes you to want snacks every time the TV is on – even if you just ate. #2 Nothing tastes right or even sounds good immediately after brushing.

Give this tip a chance. It only takes a moment and it works. Imagine how great your breath will always smell. Plus, how healthy your teeth and gums will become.

#48

FACT
If you are ordering something for shaping up you've seen on T.V., you're not gonna use it or you wouldn't have been sitting around watching T.V. in the first place.

What? It's true.

If you have time to watch T.V. you have time to workout – no debate. And don't even try to give me that whiney baby excuse about needing your "down time." Working out is the best way to de-stress and get your mind off of work or whatever it is that is bothering you. AND, working out kicks in those endorphins which make you happy – if you want to be or not.

So turn off the T.V. and get physical for at least 30 minutes. You'll be so happy you did.

#49

Start using all those infomercial shape up toys and videos you have in your garage or closet.

Go ahead; what are you "weighting" for?

Go ahead – go – shoo – just digging them out and cleaning them up might be enough of a workout for starters. They only work if used.

#50

Wear your bathing suit for 6 hours a day, once a week.

We're talking <u>daylight</u> hours here people.

This is a real tip, not a joke. If you do not own a bathing suit, go buy an inexpensive one. It is difficult to shape up once a year in time for swim suit season. By wearing your suit once a week you will always be faced with where you are – physically. When you go out you can put clothes on over your suit, but the clock stops. The moment you get back home, take off your clothes, start the clock again, and wear only your suit. If it's cold put on socks, a hat, and scarf or mittens. Or do something physical to get warm. If you have to go outside quickly, like to get the mail or bring up the trash cans, do it in your suit.

In the beginning, this is difficult (I mean really difficult). And as the weeks pass, you (& your family) will get used to your body and will become more motivated to get fit.

Note: I sometimes wear my suit two or three times a week. But then I live in Hawaii and have the opportunity to take the kids to the beach daily. I do not have a great body but I am happy with how it looks because I think it looks the best it can in my situation, at this time. I know it could look better and I remember that it used to look worse.

#51

Look at the bright side.
No matter how much weight you want to lose, there is someone out there who needs to lose more.

Your current weight is probably someone else's "goal" weight.

Besides, the goal is to get fit and wear a certain size. Not hit a certain weight. Stop thinking "weight" and start thinking healthy and fit.

WARNING:

You are now half way through this book. Did you ignore the first request for action? Are you snacking while you are reading this? Have you lost any ounces yet? Ok, enough with the questions. Go ahead and put the book down and go do something. You have plenty of food for thought. Get that journal and make your first plan for action. Then, go do something physical for at least 30 minutes. You'll feel better,

I promise. If you are reading this on a plane or in a waiting room, stop now and make your first plan for action on the last few pages of this book. That's why they're there.

#52

The next time a man comments on the size of your thighs, grab him around the waist (those love handles) and say "I know what you mean."

True story: When my oldest daughter was around 9 years old, she had obviously never before heard (or comprehended) the term, *love handles*. One day, we were all preparing to head to the beach, and my husband had asked her to put sunscreen on his back. When he thought she was finished, he began to walk away. With her arms outstretched at about waist level she exclaimed, "Daddy wait! I haven't done your *side stomachs* yet."

Sometimes guys need a reality check too. Men and women both store fat. Men tend to store it around the middle, back, and belly (above the belly button). Women store it in the thighs, butt, and belly (below the belly button). So why is it that men's fat is called "love handles" and women's fat is called "saddle bags"? "I declare that women's fat shall hence forth be known as *hula hips*" – all the better for shakin' it baby. And men's fat will now be known as "fat" (or side stomachs)☺. No longer will a man be able to grab his fat, smile and say, "check out my love handles." While women on the other hand, will no longer have to be depressed about their saddle bags. Now we can smile as we swirl seductively and say "like my hula hips?" What do you think? Are you with me on this?

#53

Do butt firming squeezes while waiting in line at the movies.

It's a great way to make new friends.
Or at least they may offer to buy your ticket.

Actually, you can do this while waiting in line anywhere. And, if you really get into it with full squats and squeezes, plus a little moaning and groaning, they will move you to the front of the line to get you serviced and out as soon as possible. Another benefit to doing this is it keeps the person/kid behind you from pushing their cart into you when you are waiting in line.

I know it sounds embarrassing, but if we all did it, it wouldn't be weird and we would all have hot buns in no time. OK, how about this? Let's just start with Tuesday's and Thursday's. Write your congress person and tell them to declare Tuesday's and Thursday's as "National Flex Your Buttocks in Public" days.

#54

The next time a skinny woman talks about how fat she is, tell her you noticed & were wondering how she could live with herself.

The poor thing actually just has low self-esteem and is crying out for a compliment. So be happy that you are confident with your current body and don't need to beg for compliments. Being *psychologically fit* is just as important as being *physically fit*. If you look good but do not know it – what's the point?

#55

March in place while watching T.V.

Watching TV is probably the second main reason you are overweight and out of shape. If you insist on watching TV, make it productive, and march. Most TV shows are depressing, violent, or cruel. Stop bombarding your mind with stuff that keeps you mentally unfit. Read (or listen) to a good book or go workout instead.

#56

Do sit-ups during T.V. commercials.

OK, so you are still watching TV. If you are marching in place great! If not, because you are too tired from being on your feet all day, fine. Now get on the floor and do abdominal work during every commercial. This will keep you from snacking and helps get you that killer "six-pack" (and I'm not talking beer) you so desire. If you watch a lot of TV you will have to add push-ups and leg lifts to your commercial workouts. At roughly 15 minutes of commercials per hour, you'll get in your 30 minutes of exercise after two of your night-time dramas.

#57

Wear combat boots all day- What a work out.

Or steel-toe worker boots.

Make sure you stand tall with good posture and keep your abs slightly tucked in for lower back support. Never wear your boots (or ankle weights) while doing floor work exercises (like leg lifts). The extra weight at your feet causes strain on your hip joint, lower back, knees, and ankles. It's not worth it. Injury from workouts often occurs when people think doing something to the extreme would be better than doing it the way it should be done. If you over do it and get hurt, you won't be able to work out and it will be hard to keep the weight off. Listen to your body and use common sense.

#58

Your body is the vehicle which will carry you through life.

What kind of vehicle are you?
What would you like to be?

Just like you change cars, you can change bodies. As a matter of fact, it was explained to me that because of cell renewal, we actually DO have a new body every 7 years. Some years the body we're in is better than others. Remember what makes your body ideal and begin to re-create it through restoration.

Take a moment right now and close your eyes. See yourself as a vehicle driving down the road. Do this for minute or so. Also, notice your road and surroundings. When you open your eyes, notice how you feel, what you saw, and what kind of car you were. Write it all down in your journal. (go ahead)

Now, close your eyes and imagine your ideal vehicle traveling through an ideal landscape. How do you feel now? Write that all down. Then make the analogy connections and write that down. For example, if you were an old style van with missing hub caps, it could mean you feel worn out, overweight, and don't care enough about your appearance – perhaps you feel like "why bother." Think about what your ideal vehicle means – subconsciously - and write that down too. (go ahead)

Once this is done you can begin your restoration project. Look at your frame and its potential. Avoid wanting what you do not have, like longer legs or bigger/smaller boobs. Work with your frame because it's the one you already own and it's the only one you can change. Remember it can take years of patient loving care to turn a neglected vehicle into a high performance show car. Keep thinking about what you do want, and enjoy your work in progress!

#59

Never buy the "King Size" version of any candy bar.

Even if it is on sale.

The regular size is always enough and the King Size one is unnecessary. "King Size" food goes hand and hand with a *king sized* you.

Exception: The big candy bar is OK, if and only if, you are splitting it with someone (other than your imaginary friend).

#60

It's not the pasta or potato that's fattening it's the toppings, so choose wisely.

*Because eating pasta or baked potato **without** a topping just isn't natural.*

When you start with white pasta or russet potatoes, then top them off with Alfredo, or butter and sour cream, you add insult (fat) to injury (starch). Move to half cup (if possible 1/3 cup) servings and low fat toppings. Or better yet, switch to wheat pasta and sweet or new potatoes for higher nutritional value and stay with the low fat sauces.

Red sauces are usually a better choice than crème sauces on pasta but only because a "low-fat crème sauce" is an oxymoron. I've been told that low-fat melted cheese and salsa are great on half a baked potato.

Fact: The simpler, processed, or starchy a carb is – like pasta, white bread and potatoes – the faster it digests into sugar/glucose which is pumped into your blood stream. The good news is you can help stabilize this process by adding a little fat – like butter or crème sauce – to your meal. The issue here is portion control. Eat what you love in much smaller portions.

#61

Stop eating two hours before bedtime.

This will minimize weight gain and weird dreams.

Everyone knows that eating late at night leads to gradual weight gain. So it's time to put the knowing to work. Not eating three to four hours before bedtime is too challenging, but two hours is doable.

Two hours before your bedtime, tape a piece of yarn across the entrance to your kitchen (or tie your fridge handles together) as a reminder. If you have kids, they can help with this and it will be good for them also.

When you eat then fall asleep you don't burn that converted fuel, so it turns to fat for future use (or not). And, because your brain has to stay more active to assist in digestion, it entertains itself with a montage of visual images otherwise known as "weird dreams."

#62

Eat till your full -
Not till your stuffed like an animal.

I've never known a fit and healthy person who gets stuffed at each meal.

Abundance is a way of life for Americans, and it shows in our waistlines and cholesterol levels. It's healthier to eat three smaller meals with three snacks in between. This is a new way of life and a huge undertaking. Doing this requires planning, will power, and perseverance. And, the rewards are immediately noticeable and great.

The moment you feel like you're getting full – you are! Stop eating and put the rest in a little container. When you're hungry again in a few hours you can finish it then or have it as a prepared snack tomorrow.

Make sure your between meal snacks are healthy and easy to grab and eat. Nuts, cheese sticks wrapped in turkey, veggie and fruit pieces, low-fat yogurt, and high fiber crackers with tuna are a few options. One of my favorite quick snacks is low fat cottage cheese sprinkled with some bacon bits. Have fun and experiment (like strawberries and reduced fat cream cheese), while keeping moderation and common sense in mind.

Healthy snacking around 10 am, 3 pm, and 8 pm will help keep blood sugar more stable, eliminate insulin resistance and keep you from binging on junk food. You are less likely to over eat when you are not starving before a meal.

#63

Remember, you no longer have to "clean your plate before you're excused from the table, young lady."

It is true there are starving children all over the world, but Americans overeating is not helping them.

If like me, you grew up poor, it may be hard for you to throw food out. Instead you may force down those last few bites because you hate to see food go to waste. Well, guess what, when you eat more than your body needs, it goes to waste in more ways than one. It goes to *waste* in your body as unused fuel, which in turn goes to your *waist* (and hips, thighs, & bottom).

Save those little servings as snacks for tomorrow. This is a good way to be "waist minded." And as for those starving children, find a local charity and give your time or money to help them out today.

#64

Stay in the tub after you pull the plug and fight the current.

It's time to get creative with the workouts.

Actually, in 1989 I saw a motivational speaker named Zig Ziglar. Even though getting fit was not an issue for me at the time, he said two things (about getting fit) I still remember. He said, "My idea of working out was to stay in the tub after I pulled the plug and fight the current." I thought that was hysterical. He then went on to talk about how he got in shape one mail box at a time. When he announced to his wife that he wanted to get fit, she went out and bought him some running shoes and a matching track outfit (AKA –wrinkly nylon matching jacket and pants). He told us with great theatrics about how he was out of gas by the time he jogged to the first mailbox. But because he made a promise to himself, he kept with it. Over time he began to jog past 15 mail boxes, then 30, then he stopped counting because he enjoyed what he was doing and did not like the distraction of counting mailboxes.

I share this with you because in order to have success, you need passion. You need to enjoy how you're living your life and feel good about your choices. What worked for you five years ago might not work for you today. Remember to stay flexible and do what feels like the right thing for you at this time.

#65

Salads are not the best food choice when swimming in Ranch or Italian dressing.

It has something to do with moderation ☺

Salads are great! They are low in fat, starch, sugar, and sodium – until you add the dressing. Then, you begin to negate your good deed. Salads are also an easy way to get in your five daily servings of veggies/fruits. There are plenty of tasty and yucky low-fat dressings on the market. Find a couple you like and use them with moderation. Sometimes I have a salad topped with fresh squeezed lemon juice – sometimes. As a measure, you know you used too much dressing if it floats alone in the bottom of your bowl when the salad is gone.

#66

Try a little balsamic vinegar, olive oil and season salt instead of Italian dressing.

Just shake it yourself and BAM, toss it on your salad.

When you make your own Italian dressing you have control over the flavors you prefer. Fresh dressing is so tasty you won't need as much because the flavors jump out at you. You can also make your own Ranch using low-fat buttermilk. There are plenty of good recipes for tasty dressings on the internet.

#67

Try plain yogurt instead of sour cream.

This is my sister's favorite fat fighter.

I personally think it's a stretch. However, I may suggest substitutions you find unpalatable. So, to each her own, play around with dietary improvements until you find ones you enjoy as much or even more than the original. I prefer Spam with 25% less sodium over the original. And Smart Balance® over butter or margarine.

#68

Use smaller dishes so your serving size will look bigger.

Restaurants do it to you all the time.

Restaurants know the psychology of how to make you feel when eating. Sometimes your plate will come on a metal or wooden platter to make it look bigger. They will also add garnishments (not for eating) and put your fruit in a little cup on your plate – and so on. When they set that huge plate in front of you, your mind says "geez, I can't eat all this." And that's even before you take your first bite, so now you think of that restaurant as the one that gives you a lot of food, but if you took away all the non-food stuff, you would be surprised at how little there actually is – that you still get full on. So, use this trick on yourself at home. Put your side dishes in little cups (which also helps with portion control) on your plate or use a smaller plate. The most famous trick is using an oval/oblong plate so your food looks stretched out in front of you.

If a restaurant wants you to stay a long time and order lots of food and drinks, the atmosphere will be warm, cushy, and softly lit. If they want to get you out quick – to make room for the next customer, the place will be bright and loud with hard seats. Sports bar restaurants will have lots of high tables and bar stool chairs to give you the "I'm single, party all night" feeling. Since you're never really sitting *down*, it seems like you're mingling at a big party.

At home you can do some of the same things. Relax and enjoy your meal with candlelight and nice music. If you're feeling a little depressed, play some good party music and stand at the sink and eat – dancing a bit while you do. And remember to use smaller or oblong plates.

#69

Avoid white stretch pants.

They are very depressing and out of fashion.

Stretch pants in general are out of style. Pants with a little stretch to them are in. When we refuse to purge our closet from time to time, we end up with clothes that are out of fashion – and unfortunately wear them. When we look good, we feel good, so get some clothes that are in fashion. Not all styles look good on all people so be honest with yourself and brave at the same time. You may need a second opinion for support on how good a new style (or color) looks on you. Rule of thumb: if you can't find a certain style you like anywhere – it's out of fashion.

Make sure you buy these new clothes on sale because chances are you will only have them for about two years, tops.

#70

Take the stairs.

Every calorie burned is a fat cell denied.

Every little bit helps. If you need the second or third floor of the mall, take the stairs not the elevator or escalator. Sometimes stairs are not an option, but when they are, take them. And take them at a brisk pace with a smile on your face.

#71

Park far away in parking lots.

And walk

Want to hear something crazy? There are people who go to my gym who will drive around the parking lot for five or ten minutes looking for a close space to park so they can go in and get on the treadmill. (I hope I am not talking about *you*)

Parking far away is good for several reasons. 1- It reduces the chances of door dings from other cars. 2- It keeps you safer because someone is less likely to throw you into their van out in the open. 3- Walking burns more calories than driving. 4- It saves gas. 5- It is good for the environment.

#72

Never compare yourself to someone who appears to have had cosmetic surgery.

I am neutral on the whole cosmetic surgery thing. However, I do know that as women, we tend to want what we can't have. When you see a gal who looks great due to her "upgrades," bless her and move on. You do not know her circumstances. You need to be concerned with you. If you are not happy with how you look, start doing what it takes to look better. Chances are… you're not *trying* as much as you are *wanting*.

#73

Remind yourself that those Cover girls are closer to animation than reality.

You wouldn't wish to look like Jessica Rabbit would you?

So stop being discouraged when you look at magazines or any printed material. Digital enhancements are nothing new. Although they are easier to accomplish now, they have been around for decades. Take note how the models eyes do not have red veins in them – at all! If you did not have veins, your eyeballs would dry up and fall out of your head. Now how sexy is that? You can never look like those girls because even THEY don't look like those girls.

The good news is they have started doing this to male models as well. Soon men will feel inferior because of their appearance also. Then maybe together we can begin to appreciate our looks as human beings instead of animated characters.

#74

Read labels when you shop.

Not when you eat.

Food labels have changed. Now they are more like vitamins with a recommended daily allowance called Daily Value or DV. Daily Values are based on a daily calorie intake of 2000. This may or may not accurately represent what you need.

Here are some things to be looking for:

Serving size – is it realistic

Calories – is it worth it

Fat – is it good fat or bad fat

Sodium – should be less than 10% DV

Carbs – are they simple/sugar or complex/fiber

Protein – should be around 35% DV (if you're choosing it for protein)

Fiber – 4% or more to be a healthy carb choice

Reading labels will help you make better choices. Reading labels also keeps you from falling for packaging misleaders - like fat free Red Vines. Reduced fat chips for example, do have less fat, but 30% more sodium. Think about your needs. When it comes to food labels, awareness brings you power.

Note: Take a look at the "Go Figure" page after the tips. It illustrates how reduced foods may or may not be better than the *full on* ones. The decision is yours.

#75

Never count calories or weigh food.

Who has the time or inclination?

Being aware of your caloric intake can be a good thing. But when you stop eating for the day because you are at your calorie/point limit, is wrong and unhealthy. It is so much more beneficial to choose healthy foods and workout faithfully. When you are burning the fuel, you don't have to be so paranoid about your food consumption – aware, yes, paranoid, no.

I was told by a nutritionist friend that 6 oz of meat is about the size of a deck of cards (see why you need that smaller plate). I use that as a visual to guide my portions because it is easy to do anyplace or time. When you focus on what you can't have, it seems like that's all you want. Instead, have what you want in moderation (are you embracing that word yet?).

The goal is to eat right six times a day (breakfast, snack, lunch, snack, dinner, and snack) and workout. Thirty to sixty minutes of exercise and smaller meals will put you on the track toward a fit and healthy body in record time. If you say you can't eat six times a day, then your portions are too big or fatty and you need better planning.

You are now shooting for satiety. Satiety means satisfied. I had trouble with this at first. I learned how to recognize when I was full by putting a little index card (I made) next to my plate that said "Full Yet?" It reminded me to check in with my stomach occasionally to get a reading on how it felt. I also knew I could save what I did not finish so I felt better about walking away from my meal.

Intermission

Just a friendly reminder that you are three quarters of the way through this book. Take a moment right NOW and write down *one thing* you know you can *do today* that will put you on the road to a better body. It could be mental, dietary or physical. Go ahead, do it now and get it out of the way. (I'm waiting...)

Also can I squeeze in a public service announcement?

Disclaimer: This is not advice, just food for thought.

Exercise Facts and Myths

Myth #1 *Exercise hurts and is not safe for people who are out of shape.*

Fact: Exercise simply means moving your body for **30 minutes** or more with a specific outcome in mind. Anything that breaks you into a light sweat (for 30 min or more) is considered exercise. Gardening, housework, and coaching soccer practice are all forms of exercise. It should never hurt. If it hurts, it is not exercise, it is torture. Find something you enjoy doing and you'll be up to an hour a day in no time.

Myth #2 *No pain - No gain*

Fact: If you suffer pain during or after working out, you either over did it or did it incorrectly. You should feel some achy muscles after you begin a new workout or sport. I call this discomfort "Muscular Roll Call" (MRC) and it is an important part of any fitness plan. MRC only occurs at the beginning of any new workout. As soon as the muscles know you know who and where they are, they stop calling out. Even the fittest person experiences MRC from time to time whenever they cross train or increase their workload. If you ever experience sharp, stabbing, or shooting pain during or after a workout venture, or if your aches never end - see a professional. There is a BIG difference between aches and downright pain. (remember, I do not claim to be a doctor)

Myth #3 *If working out every day is good, then working out twice a day is even better.*

Fact: NO

With few exceptions, more of a good thing is not better. When you over exercise, you do not give your body the chance to repair and renew itself. This is why you should cross train. Cross training mixes cardio workouts (like aerobics) with muscular ones (like resistance training) to achieve balance in the body. Adding yoga to your plan is highly recommended. If yoga is all you do however, you'll need to get on a bike, treadmill, or take up power walking for the heart. On occasion you'll get in two workouts a day, like when you run in the morning and then get invited to play doubles tennis that night (just imagine). You do not have to pass on that second workout. It's OK because it is cross training and not your regular routine. And you can count on a little MRC over the next couple of days.

Myth #4 *Lifting weights will make me look too muscular.*

Fact: Weightlifting will give your muscles definition but no one will call you *Arnold*. Bulky muscle is achieved by eating a strict high protein diet, lifting heavy amounts of weights in short, quick sets, and not stretching after the workout. It helps to be a man. Testosterone plays a large roll in the size of your muscular potential. Women can develop firm, strong muscles that become defined during and immediately after a workout, but for the most part, look smooth and tone the rest of the time. Getting "ripped and cut" is for the professionals or people who have hours to devote to the gym on a daily basis.

And now, back to the plan.

#76

Never go on a cruise.

I heard they are very fattening.

I've never been on a cruise but know many people who have. Actually, it seems like everybody but I have been on a cruise – but that is beside the point. I was told that if you request a cabin as far away from the main dining hall as possible, you could be walking up to 400 yards round trip at each of your meals. (walking after you eat –what a great idea) And, you'll be less likely to run over for a snack when it is such a trek. Today, some cruise lines offer "Fitness Cruises." But this is your vacation, indulge yourself. Just like you faithfully make the credit card payments after a vacation, you'll make the fitness payments as well. After all it's only one week out the year.

#77

Take a long lunch
& go miniature golfing.

You'll be more productive when you return.

It's important to break up your routine from time to time because as the saying goes, "A rut is just a grave with the ends kicked out." Getting excited about life can be challenging – you have to make it happen. Try new things (like that dance class from #39) and step out of your comfort zone occasionally. It's often easier to be brave with a friend, but sometimes secrecy is the only way you can do it. Whatever the case, you'll benefit mentally and physically when you do something different. Here are a few ideas to get you started:

Miniature golf

Country line dancing

Nature hike/walk

Bowling

Yoga

Ice/roller skating

#78

Drink up to 60 oz of water daily.

And learn to pee like a champion race horse.

Just kidding – and it's not true that people who drink their 60 oz a day have to pee more often (just longer). OK, enough with the jokes. I've read a variety of articles that claim our bodies are somewhere between 80-95% water. Regardless of the actual number, you'll have to agree that that's a lot of water running through us 24/7. It makes sense that we want to keep that water flowing, clean and fresh. Drinking water hydrates our cells and keeps our systems functioning. When you don't drink enough water, you begin to become more like a pond (scum and all) than a stream. Body odor, constipation, headaches, and fatigue are just a few of the many side affects you may experience when you choose not to drink enough water. If they could just put water in a little purple pill and have it prescribed by a doctor, more people would be properly hydrated. Sad but true.

Drinking water is difficult, I know. I NEVER used to drink water unless it was in something, like coffee. People would tell me, "try it with a bit of lemon in it" or "try it room temperature," but that only made it bitter and warm. I just couldn't stand to drink water. Then something happened. When I got pregnant with my first daughter, I switched my evening "put up your feet and relax glass of wine" to sparkling or mineral water. Even though it was only one glass a day, I noticed an immediate improvement in my skin and reduced achy ness in the morning. It was enough to motivate me into finding ways to get in those 60 oz!

Today I faithfully drink 48 – 60 oz a day. Even 15 years later, I still have to make a conscious effort to *think water* because it is worth it.

Water is nature's beauty secret. It is the true fountain of youth, and can be right in your hands if you would just choose it. My success with water came from starting small (moderation). Over time, I moved up one ounce a day by keeping a measured cup of water in the fridge. I started with 8 ounces, every time I opened the fridge I took a sip and at each meal I would drink a bit more. When I mastered that I added an ounce until I was up to 40 ounces (and I don't mean beer). By that time drinking water was easier and enjoyable. About once a week I still pay special attention to how much water I drink in a day to make sure I stay on track, although my body actually craves it now if I'm low.

You can begin right now by having a sip – go ahead, get one now. Keep water by your bed, in the car, your purse, the fridge and especially with you when you workout. Oh, and you can also get water from eating fruit – especially melons.

WARNING: Drinking too much water can be dangerous and hard on your kidneys. So don't think drinking 120 ounces a day will be twice as good. Have you been paying attention? The 60 ounces a day is just a guide. Your body knows what you need. Listen to it; ask it, it will tell you.

#79

Never say "diet".

Until you know it's Greek root meaning.

All-righty then, if you don't know by now why diets don't work, I'll tell you. Since *diet* is a way of life, unless you choose to continue to eat the way that *diet* has you eating forever, you will gain your weight back as soon as you go back to your *diet* or way of life.

As we age, our metabolism slows down. This means that sometimes we just have to eat less, not necessarily change what we eat. It's not always about the food; it's often about how we are living our life.

You are always on a *diet* (go look up that root) – what kind of life/body is your diet designed for? Imagine the body and life you desire. Now imagine what it will take to live that way. Make a plan and choose foods, activities, and attitudes that support your desired image. Now go for it.

#80

Don't tell anybody you're slimming down.

This keeps the pressure off.

In some cases you need to tell people you're changing your way of life. But sometimes people can irritate you into eating or not working out just to spite them – sad but true. So make your choices and live your life according to your plan. Obstacles, set backs and challenges are all part of life's story. How we write that story is up to us. Begin now by making yourself the heroine in your story called "life" and forget about the happy ending, give it a happy *now*.

#81

Put the alcohol in the meal not on the table.

A little wine sauce is better than a full glass.

I remember one summer in college, we hollowed and carved a watermelon into a basket and filled it with melon balls. Then we poured a liter of vodka over the fruit and took it to a picnic. I don't remember much after that. This story illustrates a perfect example of lack of common sense and moderation. Alcohol can give food wonderful flavor and has reduced calories when the alcohol is burned off during cooking. Experiment and create some exciting dishes that can put the fun back into eating at home. Take an extra moment to "present" your food and psychologically improve your meal. Beautifully presented food is eaten slower which allows for easier digestion and better satiety. I recently learned what a "sprig" is and now, use them often.

#82

Remember, your dress size has nothing to do with the size of your heart.

Allow your appetite for life to be a grand one.

A lot of truly wonderful women do not feel good about themselves because they are overweight. This is sad. It is easier to get fit when you truly love and admire yourself. Loving yourself is not to be confused with conceit. Conceit is when you have to go around telling people how great you are because deep down – you're afraid they won't notice. Loving yourself means you *know* how great you are and that others will know too, just by being in your presence.

Here are some ways to increase your love for your self:

1. Imagine you are to be presented with some great award. Now go to your journal and write up an introduction for yourself that will be read at the ceremony. If you just can't

think of anything stellar, ask three people you love to write one for you. Tell these people the name of your award and that it is for your journal. Then, anytime you need a loving boost – and we all do from time to time – read the introduction(s) out loud to yourself in the mirror. This is soooo fun, so do it, please – I'm begging you!

2. Each night when you get into bed, rattle off a list of things you accomplished that day that showed love for yourself and/or others. Stuff like, "I went to work, made the kids lunches, and held the elevator for a stranger" are good for starters. You may think these are things you *have to do,* but imagine what would happen if you quit doing them (and you could if you chose to). Think about your whole day from beginning to end. Remember compliments you gave, how you made someone laugh or smile, even if you drove with courtesy. This process should take at least three minutes. Then you can fall asleep with a smile on your lips and feeling good about yourself because it is the truth of who you are. If you have kids, do this with them. They'll say some of the coolest things to warm your heart.

3. Say "NO" and feel good about it. As women, we tend to want to care for others more than ourselves. This leads to personal stress and anxiety as we try to hard to make others happy. Yes, it feels really good to help others and yes, it feels really good make others happy. But not at the expense of stress to ourselves and especially not when the person we are trying to please is a "taker" or impossible to please. If you want to be happy, you need a little give and take. Stop being selfish and allow others to feel happiness too by giving them the chance to do something for you. Please say the following statement out loud and fill in the blank. "It would make me really happy if_____ _____" There, that wasn't so bad – was it? Now go say it to someone who can do it for you.

#83

If it's white, don't eat it.

Unless of course it's tofu.

Stop getting smart with me by coming up with exceptions to this rule. This is just a simple reminder for you to watch out for refined, bleached, or processed starches. Rolls, potatoes, sugar, pasta, crackers, and rice, all in the white form have little nutritional value. Nearly any food that is white has a colored counterpart that is better for you. Begin to make your life more colorful by passing on the white stuff.

#84

Keep it out of the wagon.

As they say in Hawaii.

Or keep it out of the cart. If you do not buy it, you will not be eating it. Why suffer the exercise of will power at home when you can just choose not to get it at the store in the first place. I don't buy cheese puffs for this simple reason, if the bag is open – the bag is empty. We all have food weaknesses. By not having them available, you can put temptation aside and make fit food choices instead. The next time you are at the grocery store say this little chant over and over again – "I make fit food choices because they look so good on me!"

#85

Get comfortable with boxing.

Your leftovers, that is.

You should usually have leftovers when dining out. Even if it looks like not enough to take home, have them box it up anyway. Stop being embarrassed about taking home the food you paid for. If you were at the grocery store and everything didn't fit nicely into the bags, would you say "oh that's ok, just leave it, I don't need to take it home"? of course not. The point is, when we dine out, we tend to over eat because the food is so good or we are socializing and keep nibbling because it is still in front of us. As soon as you begin to feel full, ask your food server to box it up for you. You'll be so happy tomorrow when you don't have to fix yourself something because it is already made and waiting for you.

I don't like the tactic I heard about having half of your meal boxed up as soon as it arrives. This seems like a punishment – to me – and, it puts a damper on the socializing, but if it works for you, great. Perhaps instead you can use the little card you made that says "Full Yet?" Remember, if you are riding with someone else or you had the fish, it may not be polite to stink up the car with your leftovers. As always, use your best judgment.

#86

Don't buy cream cheese with *half* the calories then use *twice* as much.

In order to *stay fit* you will also have to *think fit*. Fit thoughts include encouragements, motivation, and supportive common sense.

#87

Remember, if you only *lose* weight, you might *find* it again.

Just say "no" to the yo-yo – again

Losing weight is no longer your thing, getting fit is. Getting fit involves a plethora of activities, and going on a diet is not one of them. A fit body includes eating right and working out. A fit mind includes saying nice things to your self, about yourself. And a fit attitude includes loving where you are in life at this moment in time. Getting fit starts with a healthy attitude, not eating less or weird.

#88

Remember, diets don't work.

If they did, no one would be overweight.

If this is not making sense to you yet, go back and read the forward and introduction again. You now know that "diet" means *how* you choose to eat as much as if not more than *what* you eat. Being aware of your food options helps you make decisions about how to make fit food choices. Again, think *fit* not *thin*.

#89

Eating dry toast & half a grapefruit for breakfast will not make you thinner, only grouchy.

Just one more reason why diets don't work.

After not eating for ten or more hours, your body needs fuel. Think about keeping your system stable by having a protein, fruit, and complex carbohydrate. Breakfast proteins include meats, eggs, cheese and nuts. Breakfast fruits include jam, juice, and smoothies. Healthy breakfast carbs include breads and cereals with 4 or more grams of fiber, steel cut oatmeal, and mushrooms.

Since fruits are simple carbohydrates, eat them in small portions. Jam on toast is a double dose of carbs that will leave you feeling hungry in a very short time. Adding a slice of Canadian bacon or scrambled egg to that breakfast will stabilize insulin resistance by metabolizing the conversion of those carbs into glucose. Too much sugar/glucose in the bloodstream causes the high/low effect. While a protein only breakfast makes it harder to get in your daily doses of fruits and veggies. If you make your own smoothie, use low-fat yogurt and add some powered whey protein to help with digestion.

If you don't like to eat breakfast foods, try a small smoothie and multigrain crackers with a bit of Laughing Cow® cheese on them, or a bran muffin with a spread of reduced fat cream cheese.

#90

If you're not doing it for yourself - don't do it.

Remember the bit about loving yourself?

If you are morbidly obese – so fat it is killing you, literally, then perhaps you could be doing this because you want to see your children grow up or you don't want your loved ones to have to worry any more. But even then, it is about how **you** feel. Other people can support, and encourage you on your quest to become fit, but it is really all about **you**.

So wave your own flag and root your self into looking and feeling like a winner. Truth be told, you are already a winner if you believe it or not. Start believing, right now this very moment – go ahead, bust into song and dance about how great you are…is that *we are the champions* I hear?

#91

If someone asks if you're losing weight, tell them thank you for noticing.

And that you no longer believe in diets.

Sometimes people may ask if you've lost weight when you haven't. This is simply a compliment to which you reply, "I don't think so but thanks for the compliment." Then, revel in the fact that you obviously look good today – and remember that outfit! Quite often, when you are confident about where you are in life, you stand taller. Good posture will always make you look thinner. Aligning your bones and muscles is the cornerstone to looking and feeling fit. Show your pride in yourself by sitting and standing tall all the time.

You can improve your attitude and banish the blues by using good posture and putting a smile on your face anytime. Go ahead, try it now. Sit up straight, smile and look around slowly. Feel better? Of course you do! If you do not, it is because you did not do *all three things*, sit up, smile and look around. And if you want a bonus, add a pageant wave – it so works.

#92

Only eat fast food
if you walk there - quickly.

Otherwise, it's fat food.

Fear of million dollar litigation, has led most fast food places to put some healthier foods on their menu. If possible, choose the healthy stuff. If not, order the kids meal (smaller portions) or get your burger bun-less and share some fries. Having water instead of soda is a great fit choice in an unfit situation. When *everyone* is starving, and you're on the road, fast food is better than hurting someone (if you know what I mean).

I got my kids to quit asking for fast food by offering them the $3 instead. The only catch is, when we get home they have to help me throw something together to eat – quickly. Little ones often want the commercial "landfill toy" more than the meal. Offer to take them to the dollar store where they can pick out any TWO things they want instead.

#93

Try to eat foods that can remember where they came from.

(not so processed)

This is an ongoing challenge for me. Eating fresh means fewer, smaller trips to the store during the week. When I grew up, it was nine miles to the closest grocery store, so quick jaunts were not practical. I still have the habit today of taking one big trip and making it worth while by buying in bulk.

It is best to buy about 3 days meals at a time. Fruits and veggies have the highest value when eaten ASAP not after they sit in the crisper for a week or more. Remember to ALWAYS wash them before you put them away. That way they will be ready to eat the moment you want them. Even if the bag says "triple washed" wash it.

Homemade meals usually have greater nutritional value, but take time, so do as much preparation in advance as possible. Since you're not watching TV you should have about two hours a night – or one if you are working out in the evening – to plan and prepare your meals. Meats that are marinated not only taste better but will stay fresh longer because of the salt in most marinades.

This is also a great opportunity to practice that delegation technique mentioned earlier. Have others do the prep for you while you check in on them like a supervisor. And just in case you were wondering, meals made/heated at home from a container or box are not *homemade*. From *scratch* is more the concept we're talking about. (pasta excepted)

#94

Only allow yourself to eat healthy/organic foods while driving.

Besides, isn't it against the law to eat while driving anyway?

We are all busy, busy, busy. This often forces us to have meals in the car. Just because it's quick and on the fly doesn't mean it has to be junk/fast food. It helps A LOT to have fit snacks in the car all the time. Fruit leathers, beef jerky, nuts and "protein bars" are a few of our favorites. Of course you already have bottled water in the car – right? When you are starving and don't think you can make it home and cook something, a snack high in protein or fiber can save your life.

If you have kids who insist they are starving to death and would you "pleeeease" take them to some fast food joint, offer them the car snacks. If they decline the snacks, they are obviously not starving to death. If *you* are too hungry to have patience or think straight, make it a microwave night and heat leftovers for dinner when you get home. Do this often enough and even your kids will help you plan the day better in an effort to avoid leftovers. You can also put an end to fighting over who's getting which car snack by *dictating* who gets what – no debate. And when there is only one of some snack that of course everyone has to have, the rule is simple, mom gets it.

#95

Never call yourself a pig.

This only adds to the problem.

Getting down on yourself will only slow your progress. We all over eat occasionally. The goal is to make those occasions farther and fewer between. It is so much better to think of ourselves as a fueled up vehicle and make a plan for how we are going to burn that fuel. If you over eat, just add in a bonus workout somewhere, somehow. "This lady has just cleaned her plate and then some. Johnny, tell her what she's just won. Right you are Alex, she just won (drum roll...) a bonus hour of physical activity! (crowd goes wild).

Because our focus is on loving ourselves, name calling is **no longer an option**. Over eating is not a loving action. Remember to keep balance in all areas of your life.

#96

Instead of having a "shake", do the shake for 20 min.

And get better results.

When it comes to getting fit, there is no substitution for physical activity. I really hate to use the word exercise. It sounds too much like what they do to a demon possessed person. I like the saying "move it or lose it." But be careful you don't "shake it till you break it." Experiment around until you find something you truly enjoy doing. Remember to cross train, which means you will actually need to find two or three things you love. I love softball, but during the rainy season I use my "Turbo Jam" DVD. I hate to stretch, so I mix up the various Yogas and Pilates instead.

Give everything you try a fighting chance. Giving up on something after the first try so you can say, "oh I tried that – it didn't work for me" is a cop out. After all, I'll bet you didn't like beer or wine the first time you tried it – but now look at you ☺ OK, the point is that some things have to grow on you.

#97

Taking a pill for weight loss is like saying "I don't want a job - just give me some money."

ouch

I can say that only because I care about you. I know, you know, this is not the way to go about it. Steady and slow is the way to go. Make a plan, think fit and healthy, and earn that body you so desire one calorie and abdominal crunch at a time. Fit and trim is a way of life – not a drug.

#98

If what you need is within a half mile from your home,

WALK!

We are always in such a rush with not enough time in the day that we sometimes forget to stop and look at how we could be saving time. When something like the post office, video store, or whatever is close enough, you can get your daily workout in by walking your errands. So the next time you say, "I'm going to run to the store" literally walk there instead.

Not to mention the fact that you will save gas, keep the miles down on your leased car, and reduce pollution. That makes for five things accomplished with one action – wow.

#99

Go to the mall and shop till you drop.

Even if it's just window shopping.

My husband can't understand how my teenage daughter and I can go to the mall for three or four hours and come home with nothing. He threatens to follow us one day to see what we really do. He'll be disappointed with the truth.

When you shop till you drop make sure you wear tennies (not your fitness shoes), jeans and a button down shirt. This will help burn more calories because it takes more energy to change every time you try on something. Remember to park far away in the parking lot. When you sit down for lunch, make a fit and healthy food choice. And don't buy anything you can't afford to pay cash for. I like to "visit" clothes I want until they go on sale – because everything goes on sale.

#100

Fire the maid.

Cleaning burns lots of calories.

You could also get a part time job as a maid and make money while you workout – OK maybe not. When you clean, make sure to do it at a brisk pace with loud motivating music on that helps keep you moving.

Disclaimer: Although I only have my house professionally cleaned twice a month, I would never actually fire my maid. I love Gloria; she is worth her weight in diamonds!

#101

Fire the gardener.

Yard work is a killer workout.

Actually, I wouldn't know. I've never cared for gardening. Although I do have memories (not fond) of doing yard work as a kid – weeding a never ending back yard and pushing a non-motorized lawn mower.

If you enjoy being outside and having you hands in the earth, you can add gardening to your list of weekly workouts. All that bending, pulling, squatting, and pushing, makes for a great cross training experience.

Bonus:

Take the cat for walk then, give it a bath.

The End

Okay, you've read all 102 tips, now what? I hope with all of my heart and soul you have written at least one thing down that you've committed to do which will put you on the first step of your journey.

Ideally, you are to pick ONE thing a week to work on. If it takes a little longer to master it, that's okay, just wait to add another action on your list until you are ready. As you add things on, you will CONTINUE to maintain mastery over the previously chosen tasks. This way, by the end of a year, you will have improved the quality of your life by at least 40 actions!

It should be easy to see and imagine how improved you will look and feel. By cutting out bad food and lifestyle habits, *one at a time*, and adding beneficial physical and mental activities, *one at a time*, you are taking yourself successfully forward, step by step. Over time, the new actions will become you, and you them. This means that they no longer require much effort or thought. They are just a part of how you now choose to live your life. The future will bring change, and with it the opportunity to adapt things on your action list of things to master.

Taking the first step requires the most effort. It's like diving into the pool when you think it might be cold. True, it may be a bit uncomfortable at first, but as you get the playing and splashing around, it feels great, it makes you happy, and you wonder what all the fuss was about in the first pace.

Because things change, you are welcome to visit my website and read the monthly updates. Go to www.MindBodyLanguage. com and click on Chocolate Cake.

Thank you for sharing your time with me.

Go Figure

The food labels or Nutrition Facts found on packaging can be confusing and deceiving. Begin with looking at the serving size. For example, many cookie packages list the serving size as two (2) cookies, so I have to double everything the Nutrition Facts say because I almost always eat four (4) cookies at a sitting. Most of the time, if the label claims "reduced fat," it has higher sugar and/or sodium. It's up to you to read the labels before you buy and decide for yourself, "Is it worth it? Here are just a few examples:

Triscuit®

Nutrition Facts	Original	Low Sodium	Reduced Fat
Serving size	6	6	7
Calories	120	130	120
Calories from fat	40	40	25
Total fat	4.5g	5g	3g
Saturated fat	0.5g	0.5	0g
Polyunsaturated	2.5g	2.5g	1.5
Monounsaturated	1g	1g	0.5g
Sodium	180mg	50mg	160mg
Total Carbs	19g	19g	21g
Dietary Fiber	3g	3g	3g
Protein	3g	3g	3g

Lays® Potato Chips

Nutrition Facts	Original	Baked
Serving size	about 15 chips	about 15 chips
Calories	150	120
Calories from fat	90	25
Total fat	10g	3g
Saturated fat	3g	0.5g
Sodium	180mg	210mg
Total Carbs	15g	21g
Dietary Fiber	1g	2g
Sugars	0g	3g
Protein	2g	2g

Frosted Flakes

Nutrition Facts	Original	1/3 Less Sugar
Serving Size	¾ cup	1 cup
Calories	120	120
Sodium	150mg	180mg
Total Carbs	28g	28g
Dietary Fiber	1g	-1g
Sugar	12g	8g
*Other	15g	20g
Protein	1g	1g

*What the heck is other?

Fit Foods

Since you "wear" what you eat, I made a list of **Precious, Semi-precious**, **Rhinestone**, and **Unfit** foods for your consideration.

(Please remember, I am not a dietician – this is just "food for thought")

Precious foods are higher in nutritional value, lower in calories/fat, and better for digestion. Remember to keep the starch serving smaller and the veggie serving bigger.

Meats/Fish	Fruits – fresh	Veggies - fresh
Lean cuts of beef	All berries	Artichoke
Skinless chicken breast	Grapefruit	Asparagus
Turkey	Lemon	Alfalfa sprouts
Fish	Watermelon	Bell Peppers
Canned tuna in water	**Nuts**	Bean sprouts
Canadian bacon	Peanuts -plain	Broccoli
Turkey lunchmeats	Pecans	Cabbage
Cheese	Pistachios	Cauliflower
American – low fat	Walnuts	Celery
Cheddar – reduced fat	**Starch**	Cucumber
Feta	Brown rice	Eggplant
Mozzarella	High fiber bread	Lettuce family
Parmesan	High fiber cereal	Mushrooms
Provolone	Sourdough bread	Peas
Ricotta	Steel cut oatmeal	Spinach
String	Wheat pasta	Turnips
		Misc
		Mineral/Sparkling water
		Soy Milk

Semi-precious foods have more naturally occurring fats and sugars. You can eat these daily when you keep an eye on portion size.

Moderation is the key to success with Semi-precious food choices.

Meats/Fish	Nuts	Misc
Brisket	Almonds - raw	Milk – low fat
Wings & Legs	Pine	Salsa
Lean lunchmeats	**Starch**	Yogurt – low fat
Pork cuts	Bran muffins	Olives
Shellfish	Spinach tortillas	Pickles
Cheese	Wheat pita	Peanut butter- reduced
Jack	Wild rice	Hummus
Colby	**Veggies - fresh**	Egg salad
Cottage cheese	Avocado – 1/4	Chickpeas
Swiss	Beets	
Fruits – fresh	Carrots	
Apples -all	Tomatoes	
Mango	Yams	
Apricots		
Peaches		
Pears		
Plumbs		

Rhinestone foods are the highest in naturally occurring fats and sugars. These are the foods you fall back on when you have a craving. They are not unfit foods but can make your figure look "gaudy" if eaten daily. Use these foods to add occasional variety to your menu options.

Meats/Fish	Starch	Misc
Bacon – low salt	Corn tortillas	Half & Half
Corned Beef	English muffin	Milk
Duck	Matzo	Yogurt
Honey baked ham	Cream of wheat	Angel food cake
Pastrami	Wheat buns	Ovaltine®
Veal	**Fruits – fresh**	Semi-sweet chocolate
Cheese	Banana - half	Ice cream - reduced
Brie	Cantaloupe	Gelato
Cream cheese	Honey dew	Tapioca
Muenster	Kiwi	Baked chips
Laughing Cow®	Oranges	Popcorn - lite butter & salt
Nuts	Pineapple	Carrot cake
Brazil	All fruit juice	Banana nut bread
Cashews	**Veggies - fresh**	Raw sugar
	Corn	
	White/New potatoes	

Un-fit foods are those with very little naturally occurring nutrition. Many of these are "comfort foods." The sooner you can eliminate these from your *daily diet*, the sooner you can become fit and trim. Notice I said *daily diet* – not forever. Many of the items on this list can become "fun food." Fun foods are those you have on occasion and thoroughly enjoy them when you do. Be aware of which foods are addictive (for me it's chips) and hard to stop eating once you have had just one serving.

Un-fit foods	
Refined breads/Buns/Rolls	Instant rice white/flavored
Most breakfast cereals	Colas/Soda
Movie theatre "butter"	Macaroni salad
Cookies	Potato salad
Flour tortillas	Most pastries
Instant oatmeal	Most desserts
White rice	Whipped cream
Risotto	Alcohol
Russet/Red potatoes	Fast food
Chips	Most candy bars
Cream	Most candy
Chocolate milk	Diet Drinks
Frozen meals	Coffee drinks
Boxed side dish pastas	Energy drinks

Things to Know

Greek root for diet: way of life

Calorie: an expenditure of energy

Metabolism: the rate at which you burn calories

Glucose: naturally occurring sugar

Satiety: enough

Insulin resistance: when the glucose can't get into the muscle cells to be used for fuel, it remains in the blood which creates a variety of problems.

Glycimic Index: measures how sugary a food is

Good fats: monounsaturated like canola oil, omega-3, polyunsaturated fats found in nuts

Bad fats: saturated, the polyunsaturated - trans fat, fatty meat cuts

Endorphins: a naturally occurring chemical that helps you feel happy and energized

Resting heart rate: heart rate taken for 60 seconds while lying down, first thing in the morning. For best results count pulse for one minute, five days in a row, and average.

 Karvonen Formula: for finding training heart rate

220 - Age = Maximum Heart Rate
Max Heart Rate - Rest. Heart Rate x Intensity + Rest. Heart Rate = Training Heart Rate

Heart rate guidelines: For maximum intensity during a workout.

Beginner or low fitness level . . .50% - 60%
Average fitness level . . . . 60% - 70%
High fitness level . . . . 75% - 85%

Moderation Rule: Eat till you feel satiety or when in doubt, use common sense. (*Too much* is your arch enemy)

Suggested Reading

The following books are not suggested for the "diets," meals, or recipes. They are suggested for the LEARNING and KNOWLEDGE they provide.

Eating Well for Optimum Health
by: Dr. Andrew Weil

Eat Right 4 Your Type
by: Dr. Peter J. D'Adamo

The South Beach Diet
by: Dr. Arthur Agatston

The following books are reading I have enjoyed on my quest for a healthier mind and spirit.

Quantum Healing
by: Dr. Deepak Chopra

The Game of Life & Other Works
by: Florence Scovel Shinn

Voices of Selves
by: Dr. Carol Adams

First Things First

Because where you're headed is more important than how fast you're going.
by: Dr. Stephen Covey

See You at the Top
by: Zig Ziglar

I also recommend the following movie (DVD) about how we process information, perceive ourselves and others, and form habits.

What the Bleep Do We Know!?

The Plan

About the Author

L. Kae Graniel, the founder of Truespeak™, is a recognized key-note speaker, writer, and life coach – specializing in the 28 day Mastery Intensive. She has authored many articles for national and international magazines, newspapers and trade publications, as well as producing and hosting a variety of productions and television programs. L. Kae has a B.A. in Communication, is a Reverend, and certified Transformational Meditation™ facilitator. She has been teaching group fitness since 1984, leading over 2,500 classes in a variety of formats and environments. She is also a featured contributor and presenter for IDEA publications and their World conventions.

For more information, visit www.MindBodyLanguage.com